How to Lose Weight
And
Get a Tight Belly and Beautiful Butt

By: A.E Wilson

How to Lose Weight
And
Get a Tight Belly and Beautiful Butt

By: A.E Wilson

Table of Contents

Introduction

All over the world, there are many people who are on a daily battle to fight a physical state that has become more and more common over the passing years. Obesity and a general lack of fitness has taken over the lives of a lot of people, though only a certain number seems to be doing something to remedy the situation. Being obese or out of shape is a problem, not just because being overweight makes it hard to move around properly or fit into nice clothes, but obesity can cause other health related problems such as heart conditions and diabetes.

If you are reading this book and you want to lose weight to be healthier, feel better, or simply look good, admitting that you need to lose the weight is half the battle. Most people who are in denial are the ones who have probably tried one thing or another to lose weight, but have been let down with poor results. And who can blame them when the weight loss industry has been steadily cashing in on the hopes of overweight people to transform them overnight? It's a crime how many products or quack treatments are out there, promising to melt the pounds or take off inches just through regular usage. Other than being ineffective, some of them can be downright dangerous, with a shocking number of products proving to cause death.

The fast food industry is also one huge contributor to the growing number of obese individuals, particularly in the United States. Portions have been getting ridiculously bigger, with burgers now reaching the size of Frisbees, sodas coming in almost bucket-like containers, and small mountains of fries accompanying these meals. There are even TV shows featuring restaurants that serve extremely large portions of food, interspersed with shots of people trying to finish all of the food in front of them. If one hopes to have a flat tummy and a beautiful butt, all that food can't help to achieve that.

This book gives a realistic view about weight loss and aims to help you get a tight tummy and beautiful butt, the right way. Discover why it's hard to have a toned tummy and butt. Know all about the factors that contribute to fat. Find out when weight loss can cause harm. Also, learn all about weight loss gimmicks and why they don't work. Try out the exercises to shape your body, and learn the secrets to have a flat tummy and shapely butt. Also, read all about the facts about cellulite and how to lessen the severity of the dreaded orange peel effect on the skin. And finally, find out how to enjoy exercising and find ways to look forward to your next workout session.

There are no shortcuts to permanent weight loss and a beautiful body, but if you're willing to work for it, you can achieve it, one step at a time.

By: A.E Wilson

Chapter 1- Why It's Difficult to Have a Flat Tummy and Toned Butt

A lot of people have a hard time losing overall weight. It's even harder when weight gain is accompanied by a big and flabby tummy, a butt that is not toned, and the appearance of cellulite. Most individuals know that it will take a lot of work to improve the appearance of these areas of the body and to banish the dimpled appearance of cellulite completely. To understand what we are dealing with, we have to know why it's difficult to make a change in a fast or easy way.

If you're in a public place like a mall or the grocery, try to take a look around and find out what is the most common sign of obesity. Have you spotted it? If you said that there seems to be quite a number of people with big bellies, then that's the right answer. It is alarming how the prevalence of abdominal obesity among adults in the U.S. have increased continuously during the past 15 years. Not only are waistlines getting bigger, but along with the steady expansion of waist circumference comes the risk to certain life-threatening diseases. Some studies have even shown that waist circumference may be a better predictor for the risk of heart disease and type 2 diabetes.

Abdominal obesity has been defined as having a waist circumference of more than 40 inches for men, and 35 inches for women. Among men and women, the largest relative increase in the prevalence of abdominal obesity occurred among individuals ages 20 to 29 years old, closely followed by people who are 40 to 60 years old. To add insult to injury, the bulges around the midsection is most often accompanied by cellulite on the upper thighs and arms, and a butt that needs toning. With so many problem areas in the body, one might be overwhelmed just trying to figure out how to improve each part. But let's take a look first why it's difficult to have a tight tummy, a beautiful butt, and why it's hard to reduce the appearance of cellulite.

For instance, women who have been pregnant might find it hard to go back to their pre-baby shape. If a woman gains more than 22 pounds during pregnancy, is living a somewhat sedentary lifestyle and has not made it a habit to exercise before getting pregnant, then getting back to her slim self might be harder for her.

A person who wants to be slim and yet keeps on making poor choices on the food he eats will also have a hard time slimming down and shaping up. An unhealthy diet, one that has a lot of refined sugars and processed carbohydrates can sabotage every effort to flatten the tummy and trim the butt.

If you're expecting that infrequent exercise sessions will be enough to transform your body, know that the only way to achieve overall slimming, especially in the abdominal and posterior area, is to do exercises that will target the problem areas and to do a lot of repetitions. Doing one type of exercise such as crunches will not solve the problem since that only works the front of the abs and creates very low resistance. Same goes for only doing lunges. The muscles have to be worked in different ways to really see a difference in the way the body looks.

It may be difficult to lose the extra fat, but that doesn't mean that it's impossible to do. Making the commitment to do something about it will take a change in lifestyle, diet, and it will take some work. But in the end, it's very much worth it.

Chapter 2- The Facts About Fat

Throughout the last few decades, there have been many opinions and several findings about what causes belly fat and cellulite. Some of the information out there can be confusing or misleading, but to clarify things once and for all, here are the facts about fat and cellulite.

- **Does beer cause a fat belly?**

  There is no concrete evidence to support the idea of the beer belly. 100 ml of beer has fewer calories than the same amount of red wine, spirits and even fruit juice. It's not necessarily beer but too many calories that can turn your slim waist into a muffin top. Beer gets the reputation of being the main culprit for a big belly, when in fact, that's not the case at all. You can get fat on beer the same way as you can get fat from eating too many sandwiches, it's just that a person is more likely to drink 4 bottles of beer than eat 4 sandwiches. Think about that the next time you hang out at the local bar.

- **Are men more likely to have big bellies than women?**

  Yes. When you take in more calories than you burn, the extra calories are stored as fat. Where the body stores the fat is determined by age, gender and hormones. Young boys and girls start out with the same fat storage patterns, but puberty changes that. Women have more subcutaneous fat (the kind under the skin) than men, so those extra calories tend to be deposited in the arms, thighs and buttocks, as well as their bellies. Men have less subcutaneous fat, so they store more in their bellies.

- **Is cellulite more common among women than men?**

  Yes. If other women in your family have cellulite, there's a good chance that you will too. Cellulite is normal fat under the skin, and this fat appears bumpy because it pushes against connective tissue, and that causes the skin above it to pucker.

- **Does having cellulite mean that I'm overweight?**

  No. In fact, even thin people can have it. If you are overweight though, losing weight may reduce cellulite. Other factors that influence how much cellulite you have and how visible it is can be due to a poor diet, fad dieting, a slow metabolism, lack of physical activity, hormone changes, total body fat, dehydration, and the thickness and color of your skin. Only 2% of women don't get cellulite, and they're women of African descent.

- **Do high fat foods cause excess fat storage in the belly?**

  No. Actually, healthy, monounsaturated fats like those found in olive oil, nuts, seeds and avocados are really effective at beating belly fat. Sugar, on the other hand, accelerates fat storage.

- **Are women more likely to get a fat butt than men?**

  Yes. Women have a greater tendency than men to store fat in the lower body.

- **What foods will make me gain weight and have a big tummy and a fat butt?**

  Processed and refined carbohydrates, such as those found in breads and most cereals can make a person gain weight and have a fat butt. Saturated fats like those in French fries can do the same thing to the body, as well as fast food and soft drinks.

Chapter 3- When Weight Loss Causes Harm

Wouldn't it be nice if there was a magic potion out there that you could drink, and instantly you'd lose weight? Or just wearing something at night can magically shrink the fat around your belly? The weight loss industry makes a fortune on quick-slim claims that they make year after year. It seems like every season, there seems to be a new fad that comes along, proudly proclaiming itself to be better than the last fad. Unfortunately, true weight loss cannot be rushed. There have been a lot of products in the market, all of them promising to melt the fat and make the pounds go away in a jiffy. Some of them actually worked, but the weight loss was accompanied by side effects, some of which have actually caused a number of deaths.

Here are some weight loss methods that don't work for the long term, and proven to have negative effects on the body:

- **Crash Dieting**

  Though this may result in weight loss, it also leads to longer term weight gain. When the body is low on energy, it causes you to crave foods that are high in sugar and carbohydrates. So when you give in, you'll often eat more than the recommended serving, causing weight gain.

- **Diet Pills**

  Since the 90's the market has been flooded with all sorts of diet pills. Among the most notorious are Bangkok Pills, a slimming pill from Thailand. A packet consists of several multicolored pills, meant to be taken several times a day. The pills were found to contain phentermine, fenfluramine and ephedrine among others. Each of these substances are dangerous on their own, but when combined, they can become lethal. Those who have taken Bangkok pills have exhibited symptoms same as those who have taken crack, such as insomnia, anxiety, and loss of appetite. Though the slimming effect is immediate, the side effects such as palpitations, nausea, and chest pains were reported by majority of users. It was also reported that when people stopped taking the pills, they immediately gained back the weight they lost, plus an extra 15 to 20 pounds on top of that. In drastic cases, there have been those who had stroke, seizures, heart attacks, and death.

Another slimming pill that has dangerous side effects is the Brazilian Diet Pill marketed under the name of Emagrace Sim and Herbaslim which contains Librium, Prozac which is an antidepressant and Fenproporex. This combination of uppers and downers can cause extreme mood swings. Models who took the pill experienced extreme personality changes and hypersensitivity to touch.

- **The Clen Fat Burner**
  Clen or Clenbuterol is a steroid used to treat respiratory illnesses in horses. It is in no way approved for human use, but it made headlines last year after athletes were banned from the Pan Am games after testing positive for Clen. It is also often taken illegally by athletes and models to boost

muscle mass and trigger weight loss. Clenbuterol has never been tested on humans, and it can cause damage to the heart.

- **The K-E diet or Feeding Tube Diet**
  This involves inserting a naso-gastric tube through the nose, through which a nutrient solution with approximately 800 calories is delivered to the stomach. This diet was popularized by brides looking to drop the last 10 pounds they've been meaning to shed before the big day, although this type of diet claims that as much as 20 pounds can be shed in 10 days. This procedure also involves finding a doctor to perform the procedure.

  This type of diet is harmful to the body because there's a risk of inflammation and infection, not to mention how questionable credentials of any doctor who's willing to perform this procedure on anyone.

Chapter 4 - Weight Loss Gimmicks

So many people have been conned into buying products being touted to promote weight loss, and some of them range from the completely normal to the absurd. Some of the things out there obviously have no effect on fat loss, however, because of clever marketing tactics that taps into the hopes of many people who will do anything or try anything to be slim, these products get snapped up in a jiffy. No wonder the weight loss industry is one of the most fruitful industries during the last three decades.

When it comes to weight loss, it's important to know the things that don't yield results. Here are just some examples of gimmickry dreamed up by people to make you think that you need these things to lose the pounds:

- **Anti-Cellulite Creams and Lotions**

    You might want to read the label very carefully the next time you go shopping for the next dream cream to get rid of cellulite. No cream will get rid of cellulite, the most they can do is reduce the appearance of cellulite by firming the skin. To be able to do that, the cream has to contain caffeine, which draws the water out, leaving skin looking a bit firmer, albeit temporarily.

- **Weight Loss Lollipops**

    These lollipops, spiked with Hoodia are claiming to aid in weight loss by suppressing the appetite. However, there is no proof that these lollipops can actually deliver on that promise. It's the same principle that is applied by smokers who wish to stop smoking: to keep their mouth busy, they would chew gum or eat hard candies so that the urge to smoke would be lessened. By sucking on these lollipops for about half an hour, you forget that you're actually hungry. The mind is distracted from hunger, but you could probably have the same effect from any regular lollipop.

- **Weight Loss Sunglasses**

  One of the goofier products out there, this aims to make the wearer look at food in a new yet disgusting light, which, supposedly will quell the appetite. The glasses look like normal aviators, except that the lenses are a bright blue. Upon wearing the glasses before eating, everything you'll see will be a shade of blue, which will hopefully turn you off from consuming whatever's on your plate. There's an actual explanation to this. Color theorists say that blue is the most unappetizing color, since blue food makes us think of mold or any food that's past its expiration date. However, there's no scientific data saying that blue is the least appetizing color.

- **Ear stapling**

  Many people believe that the ancient Chinese practice of acupuncture can help to speed along the weight loss process. However, ear stapling is based on auricular acupuncture, which doesn't have any scientifically proven benefits yet, and in traditional acupuncture, the needles are placed in acu-points for a certain amount of time, then removing them before the person leaves the clinic. Ear stapling can lead to infection and can be very painful.

- **Slim Rings**

  These are flexible plastic rings meant to be worn on the big toes. According to the manufacturers, what causes the slimming effect is a small bump on the device that is positioned downwards, so each time you take a step, you shift the distribution of your weight. This causes you to stand and walk differently, forcing your body to use lesser used muscles and help you get your problem areas toned. This is supposed to make a huge difference in the appearance of a large butt and thighs. However, unnatural walking can cause posture problems and you may feel some pain in your legs after a while.

- **HCG Hormone Injections**

  Developed by Kevin Trudeau, a man with no medical training and a convicted felon, he made billions of dollars by peddling HCG shots as a cure for obesity, which is not what it is. HCG is a hormone that is found in pregnant women's urine, so basically, what you get is a syringe full of human urine.

  A good rule of thumb to follow: If it seems too good to be true, it probably is. Nothing beats a careful diet and exercise to help shape the body and help you maintain it for a long period of time.

Chapter 5- How to Get a Tight Tummy

At one point or another, you probably attempted doing numerous sit-ups or crunches in hopes of having a flat stomach. However, you're probably noticing that no matter how many sit-ups or crunches you do, your stomach still looks the same, and all you've got to show for your efforts is a recurring back pain. Doing these exercises may also cause more harm than good.

Crunches involve lying on your back and repeatedly bending and extending your spine. That causes excessive strain on your lower back, where a lot of nerves are located and is very prone to wear and tear from repetitive movements. Crunches and sit-ups also don't burn as much calories as you should to melt away the fat in your abdominal area, so here are other alternative exercises that you should try.

To flatten your tummy after giving birth:

Now that you've given birth, you're probably dismayed about the fact that your tummy is still so big and flabby. The good news is that your belly will diminish in size in a few months. The bad news is that it will still have that soft, doughy look. To solve this problem, you have to work on your transverse abdominal muscles. These muscles are connected to your back muscles and rectus abdominals, and the transverse muscles acts as a girdle to your whole midsection. These muscles lie horizontally and help keep your organs in place, and they can get very weak after childbirth.

When you're cleared by your doctor to exercise, make sure to do these moves to target the transverse muscles:

Scissor Kicks

1. Start by lying on the floor. Place your hands under your buttocks and keep your back pressed against the floor.
2. Raise one leg about 10 inches off the ground and slowly lower it back down. As you lower one leg, raise the other.

3. Do three sets of 10 repetitions.

Inverted V

1. Lie on the floor, hands under your head. Raise both legs to form a V. Then, slowly lower legs so that the knees are now touching.
2. Slowly straighten out the legs while lowering them to the floor.
3. Do three sets of 15 repetitions.

Pelvic tilts

1. Lie on the floor. With your back pressed against the floor, bend your knees, keeping your feet on the floor.

2. Slowly lift your pelvis up and hold briefly before lowering slowly back to the ground. Your upper body should remain pressed against the floor throughout the whole movement.

3. Do three sets of 15 repetitions.

Exercises to flatten the tummy and firm the abs

There are a lot of exercises designed to flatten the tummy and slim the waistline, but in order to achieve great results, one must take care to target all of the muscles groups in the stomach. The abdominals have many different parts, but they can be divided into 3 main parts which are the upper, lower, and side or oblique muscles. If all of the muscles are strong, then the whole stomach will be flat and firm. Be careful not to do any exercises that don't do anything for your abs, such as crunches, as they cause back pain. Whenever you do abdominal exercises, make sure that lower back is straight and firm to have good results and minimize the risk of injury.

For Upper Abdominals
1. Lie down on the floor. Raise your legs and rest your calves on a chair
2. Raise your chest up towards your knees. Do three sets of 10 repetitions.

1. Lie flat on the floor and place your hands behind your head.
2. Bring the knees in to the chest and lift the shoulder blades off the floor without pulling or straining the neck.
3. Rotate to the left, bringing the left elbow towards the right knee while straightening the other leg.
4. Switch sides, bringing the left elbow towards the right knee.
5. Continue alternating sides using a pedaling motion. Do one to three sets of 12 repetitions.

For Lower Abdominals

1. Lay down on your back with your legs out straight. Lift your head and neck and alternate moving your feet up and down.
2. . While doing this, make sure that you keep your head up, your knees locked, and move your feet up and down for as long as you can.
3. Do this until you can't anymore, then relax. Do two to three sets.

1. Lie flat on your back with your legs up as if you're resting your calves on a chair or a table.
2. Without moving your upper back, contract your lower abs, lift your butt off the floor and pull your knees inward toward your head.
3. When your knees are chest high, pause for 5 seconds and slowly return to starting position.
4. Do three sets of 12 repetitions.

For Side Abdominals or Oblique muscles

1. Lay on one side of your body with your back completely straight.
2.
3. Slowly crunch your legs towards your torso, while doing this, make sure that you're contracting your sides.
4. At the peak contraction point, hold it there for as long as you can. Repeat for the other side.

Do two sets of 10 repetitions for each side.

1. In a standing position, hold a dumbbell or a medicine ball above your body and to the side of your shoulder.

2. Diagonally rotate with extended arms from above your shoulder, down and across your body to the outside of your hips. While doing this, imagine that you're doing the same movement as you would if you were holding an axe and chopping wood.

3. Do two to three sets of 12 repetitions.

Chapter 6- How to Have a Beautiful Butt

For the past decade, more people have been striving to have a beautiful butt. And with muses such as Jennifer Lopez, Kim Kardashian and Jessica Alba serving as inspiration, more women have been scrambling to get the same beautiful posterior as these ladies. The ideal butt is described to be rounded, perky, and firm, with no hint of cellulite whatsoever. When asked what they would like to change about the appearance of their buttocks, 85% wanted a firmer, more rounded appearance, and 30% would like to increase the size of their buttocks, since a lot of women have flat-looking buttocks to contend with.

Unfortunately, those who seek immediate gratification have resorted to unsafe methods to get a beautiful butt. Hydrogel silicon injections have been in vogue for the past decade, until reports surfaced of men and women having adverse reactions to them which includes infection and even death. Some have even tried the Brazilian Buttock Lift, wherein fat from unwanted areas such as the abdomen, sides and back are injected into the gluteal area and sometimes the hips. Doctors who perform the surgery say that this improves the overall shape of the lower back, hips and lumbar area, although they are also quick to issue a disclaimer stating that not all of the fat that is transferred survives the procedure, and 40 to 50% of the fat transferred can shrink over time. Not only is the procedure costly, but it doesn't offer a permanent solution to the problem.

Clearly, the only way to get a beautiful butt is to eat the right kind of food and to have an exercise regimen specifically designed to target the buttocks. Here are a couple of exercises that you can do on your own to improve the appearance of your butt.

To improve a flat butt:

If you have a flat butt, the muscle fibers in your glutes need to be stimulated and engaged. Exercise moves that extend the glutes to the maximum before contraction will improve the appearance of a flat butt, making it look rounder.

Hip Raises
- Lie faceup, with knees bent, feet flat on the floor. Squeeze glutes and lift hips off the floor for three counts.
- Hold for two counts and lower hips to the floor. Do two sets of 12 repetitions.

Power Extensions
- Start on hands and knees with back straight, wrists directly beneath shoulders.
- Simultaneously extend left arm and right leg in line with body and hold for 2 counts.
- Switch sides. Do two sets of 12 repetitions.

Rear End Reach
- Stand with feet hip-width apart. Step with right foot into a side lunge so that the right knee aligns with the right foot and the left leg is straight.
- As you lunge, twist the torso and reach for the right foot with your left hand.
- Push off with your right foot to return to standing position.
- Repeat on the left side. Do two sets of 8 repetitions.

Kick butt

- Start on your hands and knees, keeping your back straight, wrists directly in line with shoulders.
- Squeeze glutes to lift right leg, and keeping knee bent at a 90-degree angle, push sole of foot towards the ceiling until hamstring is aligned with torso. Be careful not to arch your back.
- Return to starting position and switch sides. Do two sets of 12 repetitions.

To improve a saggy or flabby butt

Toning the buttocks will require a variety of exercises to target the different areas of the posterior, particularly the smaller muscles which are the gluteus medius and minimus which are along the outer thigh, and the gluteus maximus, the largest muscle in the buttocks.

Carving Curl
- Lie face down on the floor with your head resting on your folded arms.
- Squeeze a 1 pound dumbbell or rolled up towel behind your bent left knee, keeping your foot flexed. Tuck in the pelvis to flatten the back.
- Lift bent leg a few inches off the floor, then lower. Do 20 repetitions before switching sides.

Bend and Extend
- Stand in front of a chair, bend over and place hand on the seat. Your right forearm should be on top of the chair back.
- Tuck in your pelvis and extend your left leg behind you, keeping your foot flexed.
- Pulse your left leg up and down 10 times, then with your leg, trace 5 circles going counterclockwise, then 5 circles going clockwise.
- Hold the leg lift for 5 counts, then switch sides.
- Do 12 repetitions for each leg.

Swaying Bridge
- Lie faceup on the floor with your knees bent, feet flexed, keeping your heels on the floor and arms by your sides.
- Step heels out so your legs are slightly wider than shoulder-width.
- Lift your hips so that your body forms a straight line from your rib cage to your knees, then lower. Do 10 repetitions.
- With your hips lifted, sway hips from left to right as you squeeze your glutes. Do 20 repetitions.
- With hips lifted, pulse your hips up and down twenty times.

Door Hinge
- While standing, bend at hips and rest your right forearm on the back of a chair. Squeeze a rolled up towel behind your left knee, keeping your foot flexed. Place your left hand on your hip.
- Lift your knee out to the side, then bring it back towards your chest, then behind you. Do 10 repetitions.
- While your knee is behind you, do 20 pulses by moving your leg to the right by about an inch, then to the left. Switch sides and repeat.

Chapter 7- The Facts About Cellulite

A lot of women have it. Chances are, if your mother had it, you'll have it too. And only a very small percentage of women don't have it.

Cellulite... Rich and poor women have it. Overweight and yes, even thin people can have it. Light skinned women usually have it, as lighter skin is usually thinner. Studies show that 95 percent of women have a type of cellulite on their body. It is often hereditary, so if you have it, it's very likely that you are not the only one in the family who has it. Though cellulite is common enough, there's still a lot of information out there about what it really is, what causes it, and how to get rid of it. So to clear up things, here are the facts about cellulite.

Types of Cellulite:

First of all, cellulite is not a medical condition. It is fat that is found under the skin, and though it isn't dangerous to one's health, it can look unsightly.

There are three types of cellulite. Adipose cellulite is firm cellulite and causes an orange peel effect on loose skin. Oedematous cellulite is fluid retention, this is soft cellulite on loose skin. And finally, there's Fibrotic cellulite, which is hard compact cellulite with orange peel effect.

In addition to these, there are also four grades of cellulite which categorizes the severity of each case:

Grade 1- no visible cellulite, even when the skin is pinched.

Grade 2- no visible cellulite when lying down or standing. An orange peel texture will only be seen if the skin is pinched.

Grade 3- cellulite is only visible when standing, and may disappear when lying down.

Grade 4- visible cellulite when standing or lying down.

What Causes Cellulite

Aside from being hereditary, there are a lot of factors that contribute to the onset of cellulite. Going on frequent crash diets is one of these factors. Another primary factor is hormones, because the presence of too much estrogen can aggravate cellulite. Ladies live a sedentary lifestyle are also prime targets of cellulite. Diet also plays a major role when it comes to having cellulite. Refined and processed foods, artificial foods that contain a lot of sweeteners, additives and chemicals, as well as sugar and foods that contain a lot of sugar are all thought to contribute the orange peel effect.

How to Get Rid of Cellulite

Short of undergoing a medical procedure, there really is no way to get rid of cellulite completely, but there are ways to lessen the severity of the orange peel effect. One inexpensive way to do this is by body brushing. Use a dry body brush, and stroke towards the direction of the heart to improve blood circulation. A hard massage on the thighs will increase fat dispersion if done on a regular basis.

Unfortunately, no cream or lotion in the world can melt cellulite away. The most you can do is to pick a firming lotion, either with methyl nicotinate or caffeine which can dehydrate skin and reduce the amount of retained water, so skin looks firmer temporarily.

Energizing movements and warming exercises can help lessen the appearance of dimpled skin if done consistently. Running, swimming or brisk walking are all highly effective to increase blood circulation and to loosen the fat tissues.

By: A.E Wilson

Chapter 8- Attitude Towards Exercise

Most people hate the thought of working out. Who wants to get up at the crack of dawn to run a few laps? There are even some people who dread going to the gym. What causes this negative attitude towards something that is beneficial to our health?

It has been documented over and over again that regular exercise has plenty of health benefits, including lowering risks of being obese. However, only 30 percent of Americans who are trying to lose weight are meeting the National Institute of Health exercise guidelines of 300 minutes a week of exercise. Sadly, those who really want to lose weight have the tendency to feel embarrassed and intimidated about exercising. What are the factors why people will do anything to avoid exercising?

For people who don't know what to do in a gym or have no idea how fitness equipment works, they will often steer clear of fitness clubs, fearing that they'll do something that will make them look awkward or stupid in front of others. Also, most people have had bad experiences with sports and fitness. They seldom feel competent or confident playing sports or participating in any fitness activity. Also, most people are embarrassed about their bodies. They avoid any situation where their physique will be more visible to others. Like the overweight girl who covers herself up completely at the beach, most overweight people will shun working out in a gym since they know that they will have to do it in front of people.

Personal trainers who don't tailor fit the way they motivate their clients can also contribute to workout phobia. Many people have had bad experiences regarding the methods of the trainer. What works for one person may not work for another, thus if someone thrives on a strict, boot camp style of motivation, others may prefer a gentler approach.

People who choose to workout on their own may find that the lack of accountability will result to slacking off. They will often exercise less, do the exercises wrong, or just skip them altogether. It takes a lot of discipline and willpower to exercise on your own, so this method might not be apt for people who have a hard time sticking to a regimen.

Is it possible to enjoy exercising? Yes it is, but you definitely have to find the right type of exercise for you. The exercises in this book are designed to shape your tummy and butt, yet to achieve overall slimming, you must have an exercise regimen to look lean, healthy, and to keep other health problems at bay.

If you like exercising with a group of people, consider enrolling in a spinning class. It's one of the hottest trends right now, and it is fantastic for overall shaping, particularly the core and glutes. You can also try a dance class such as Zumba. You'll feel energized, and its lots of fun, as if you just went out dancing with your friends.

If you like the military or boot camp approach, you can try working out with a personal trainer. Having a good personal trainer help you with your workouts could be worth the cost, as you'll often see results faster compared to working out on your own. It can be costly, but think of it as an investment. You're investing in your health, which is better than spending your retirement fund on medication or treatments to treat obesity related diseases.

If you get bored staying in one place, a constant change of scenery while exercising is the solution. You could try biking, surfing or wakeboarding. These activities are great for targeting the glutes and the abdomen, and can minimize the appearance of cellulite.

Want something low impact? Try yoga or pilates. Both have been enthusiastically recommended by people who saw major changes in their body within weeks of doing yoga or pilates moves. You'll notice that you're slimmer, your muscles are lean and defined, not bulky, and you're more flexible and relaxed after each session.

Strapped for cash? You can take up running or jogging- all you need are some running shoes. You don't even need to shell out mega bucks to get top branded shoes. There are lots of inexpensive options out there that will work just as well. You can also try to exercise at home, substituting weights with plastic bottles of water, and there are some exercises that you can do wherein you'll only need a rolled up towel and a chair, such as those that were featured in the previous chapters.

Or you can do something you truly enjoy. A game of basketball or soccer after work can energize you and give you a full body workout. You'll have fun as you lose weight, and suddenly, exercise doesn't seem like such a daunting task anymore.

It's important that you exercise to stay fit and healthy. It's the only way to make sure that the weight stays off when you eventually lose it, and it's the safest way to reshape your body.

Make a commitment to exercise today. You can start small: Perhaps, you can take a walk for about three blocks today, then walk a little farther the next day. You could also try taking the stairs instead of the elevator. There's no time like the present, so make sure to have an exercise regimen in place. Eventually, you'll be pleased with the difference it makes, as you'll see how you become fitter and stronger than ever.

www.ingramcontent.com/pod-product-compliance
Lightning Source LLC
Chambersburg PA
CBHW070242290526
45789CB00004B/1733